THE LYMPHATIC DIET COOKBOOK

Dr. Kimberly Carlos

Copyright © 2023 by Dr. Kimberly Carlos

All rights reserved. No part of this publication may be reproduced, distributed, or transmitted in any form or by any means, including photocopying, recording, or other electronic or mechanical methods, without the prior written permission of the publisher, except in the case of brief quotations embodied in critical reviews and certain other noncommercial uses permitted by copyright law.

TABLE OF CONTENT

INTRODUCTION 7

CHAPTER ONE 11

Following a Lymphatic Diet with Benefits 11

CHAPTER TWO 15

14-Day Lymphatic Diet Meal Plan 15

Day 1 15

Day 2 15

Day 3 16

Day 4 17

Day 5 17

Day 6 18

Day 7 19

Day 8 19

Day 9 20

Day 10 21

Day 11 21

Day 12 22

Day 13 23

Day 14 24

CHAPTER THREE 25

Lymphatic Diet Breakfast Recipe 25

1. Green Detox Smoothie.. 25

2. Overnight Chia Pudding 25

3. Veggie Omelette 26

4. Greek Yogurt Parfait... 27

5. Quinoa Breakfast Bowl.. 28

6. Berry and Spinach Smoothie Bowl....................... 29

7. Avocado Toast with Poached Egg......................... 29

8. Berry Protein Pancakes....................................... 30

9. Peanut Butter Banana Smoothie 31

10. Fruit and Nut Oatmeal 32

Lymphatic Diet Lunch Recipe 33

1. Lymphatic Detox Salad.. 33

2. Lentil and Vegetable Soup.................................... 34

3. Chickpea and Avocado Wrap 35

5. Mediterranean Tuna Salad 37

6. Turkey and Vegetable Stir-Fry 38

7. Spinach and Quinoa Stuffed Bell Peppers 39

8. Grilled Salmon Salad 40

9. Sweet Potato and Lentil Bowl........................ 40

10. Quinoa and Kale Bowl with Lemon-Tahini Dressing
.... 41

CHAPTER FOUR.. 43

Lymphatic Diet Dinner Recipe 43

1. Baked Salmon with Garlic and Herbs..................... 43

2. Quinoa-Stuffed Bell Peppers 44

3. Lymphatic Detox Soup 45

4. Grilled Chicken with Lemon-Garlic Asparagus 46

5. Lentil and Vegetable Stir-Fry 47

6. Lemon and Herb Quinoa with Roasted Vegetables .. 48

7. Spinach and Kale Salad with Grilled Shrimp 49

8. Turkey and Vegetable Stir-Fry 50

9. Mediterranean Tuna Salad 51

10. Grilled Veggie and Quinoa Bowl 52

Lymphatic diet snacks recipe 53

1. Mixed Berry Smoothie 53

2. Cucumber and Hummus 54

3. Greek Yogurt with Berries 54

4. Sliced Apple with Almond Butter 55

5. Carrot and Celery Sticks with Hummus 55

6. Trail Mix 56

7. Sliced Bell Peppers with Guacamole 57

8. Cottage Cheese with Sliced Peaches 57

9. Nut Butter and Banana Wrap 58

10. Caprese Skewers 58

CONCLUSION 61

INTRODUCTION

Once upon a time in a small town nestled among rolling hills, there lived a woman named Sarah. Sarah had always struggled with her health. She felt tired all the time, had swollen limbs, and her skin seemed to constantly break out. Doctors couldn't provide her with a definitive diagnosis, and she grew frustrated as her health deteriorated.

One day, while browsing the internet in search of answers, Sarah stumbled upon a blog post about the lymphatic diet. It promised to detoxify the body, reduce inflammation, and boost the immune system. Intrigued, Sarah decided to give it a try.

The lymphatic diet required her to eliminate processed foods, dairy, and gluten from her meals. Instead, she filled her plate with fresh vegetables, fruits, lean proteins, and plenty of water. She also started incorporating lymphatic-boosting foods like ginger, garlic, and leafy greens into her daily routine.

The first few weeks were challenging as Sarah adjusted to her new way of eating, but she persevered. Slowly but surely, she began to notice changes. Her energy levels increased, her skin cleared up, and her limbs no longer felt heavy and swollen. It was as if a fog had lifted from her life.

As time passed, Sarah continued to follow the lymphatic diet faithfully. She also started practicing yoga and gentle exercises to stimulate her lymphatic system further. Her health continued to improve, and she even shed some excess weight along the way.

Sarah's transformation was nothing short of remarkable. Her friends and family couldn't believe the difference in her appearance and vitality. She became a beacon of hope for others in her community who were struggling with similar health issues.

Through her journey with the lymphatic diet, Sarah not only regained her health but also found a new purpose. She started a local support group to help others embrace this dietary lifestyle and experience the same transformative effects.

In the end, Sarah's story became an inspiration to many, proving that sometimes the simplest changes in our diet and lifestyle can lead to profound improvements in our health and well-being.

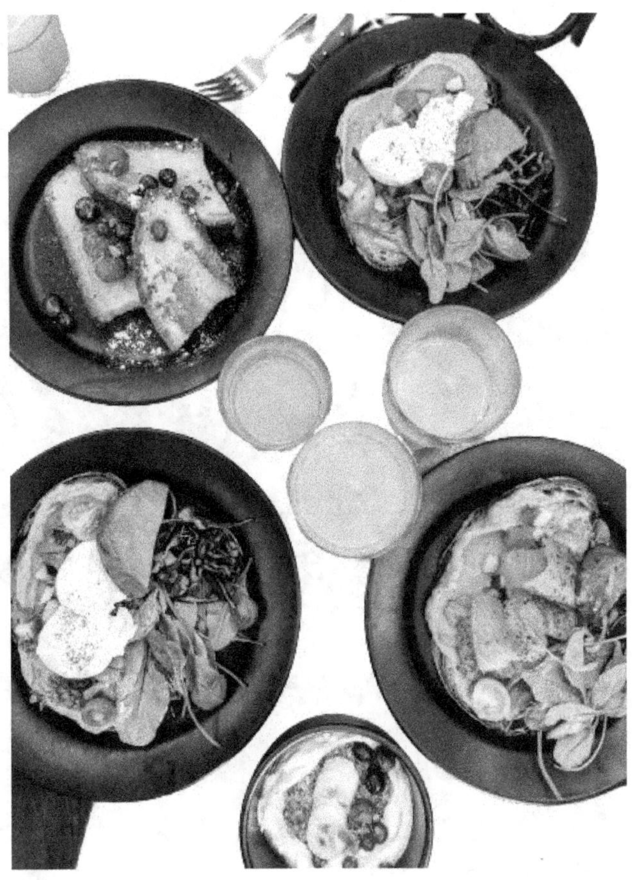

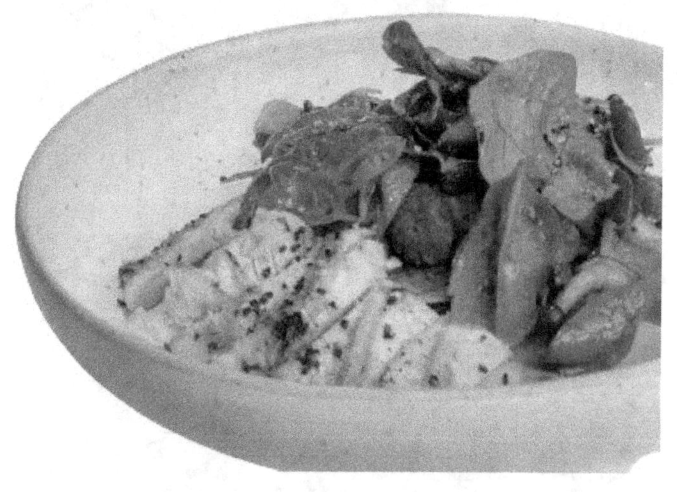

CHAPTER ONE

Following a Lymphatic Diet with Benefits

Following a lymphatic diet can offer several health benefits, including improved detoxification, reduced inflammation, and enhanced immune function. Here's a guide on how to follow a lymphatic diet with its associated benefits:

1. Consult a Healthcare Professional: Before making any significant dietary changes, consult with a healthcare professional or a registered dietitian. They can provide personalized guidance based on your specific health needs and goals.

2. Increase Hydration: Proper hydration is essential for a healthy lymphatic system. Aim to drink plenty of water throughout the day to help flush toxins from your body and keep your lymphatic system functioning optimally.

3. Emphasize Whole Foods: Focus on whole, unprocessed foods that are rich in nutrients. Include plenty of fresh fruits, vegetables, whole grains, and lean proteins in your diet. These foods provide essential vitamins, minerals, and antioxidants that support overall health.

4. Reduce Inflammatory Foods: Minimize or eliminate foods that can contribute to inflammation, such as processed foods, sugar, refined grains, and excessive saturated fats. These can impede lymphatic function and overall health.

5. Include Lymphatic-Boosting Foods:

- Incorporate foods known to support lymphatic health, such as ginger, garlic, onions, and leafy greens. These contain compounds that can stimulate lymphatic flow and reduce inflammation.
- Eat fruits like citrus, which are rich in vitamin C, a powerful antioxidant that supports the immune system.

6. Limit Dairy and Gluten: Some lymphatic diets recommend reducing or eliminating dairy and gluten because they can contribute to inflammation in some individuals. However, it's important to consult a healthcare professional before making such dietary changes.

7. Practice Mindful Eating: Slow down and savor your meals. Chewing food thoroughly can aid digestion and help your body absorb nutrients more effectively.

8. Incorporate Herbal Teas: Certain herbal teas like dandelion root or nettle can help promote lymphatic drainage and overall detoxification. Enjoy them as part of your daily routine.

9. Engage in Physical Activity: Regular exercise, especially activities like yoga, rebounding, or deep breathing exercises, can help stimulate lymphatic flow and improve circulation. Find an exercise routine that you enjoy and can maintain consistently.

10. Stay Consistent: Consistency is key when following a lymphatic diet. Gradual changes in your dietary habits are more sustainable and can lead to long-term benefits.

11. Monitor Progress: Keep a journal to track your energy levels, skin condition, and any other health improvements you may experience. This can help you assess the effectiveness of the diet for your specific needs.

12. Adjust as Needed: Be open to adjusting your diet as your body's needs change. Listen to your body, and if you experience adverse effects or don't see the desired benefits, consult with a healthcare professional to make necessary modifications.

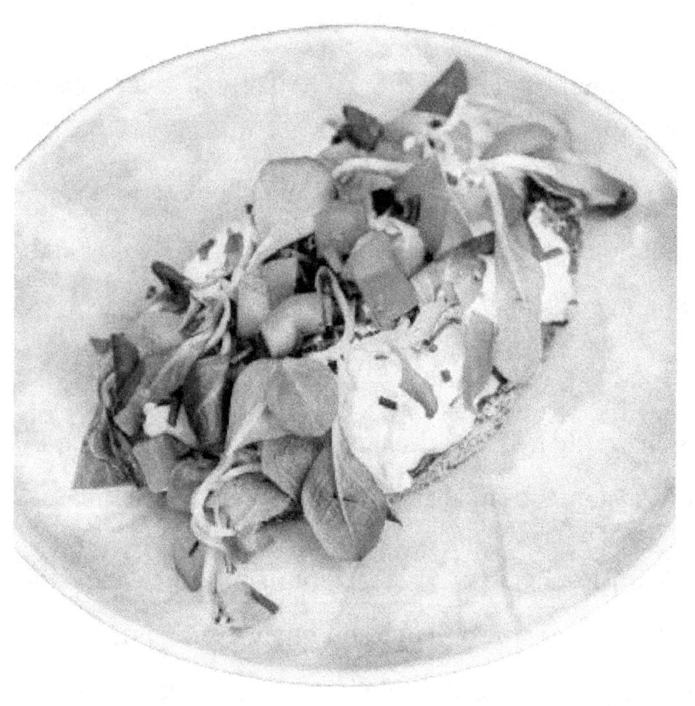

CHAPTER TWO

14-Day Lymphatic Diet Meal Plan

Day 1

Breakfast:

- Green smoothie with kale, spinach, banana, and chia seeds.

Lunch:

- Grilled chicken breast salad with mixed greens, cherry tomatoes, cucumbers, and olive oil and lemon dressing.

Dinner:

- Baked salmon with steamed broccoli and quinoa.

Snack:

- Carrot and celery sticks with hummus.

Day 2

Breakfast:

- Greek yogurt with berries and a sprinkle of flaxseeds.

Lunch:

- Lentil soup with a side of mixed greens.

Dinner:

- Stir-fried tofu with bell peppers, broccoli, and brown rice.

Snack:

- Sliced apples with almond butter.

Day 3

Breakfast:

- Oatmeal topped with sliced bananas and a drizzle of honey.

Lunch:

- Quinoa and black bean salad with diced avocado, cherry tomatoes, and cilantro dressing.

Dinner:

- Grilled shrimp with roasted asparagus and sweet potato.

Snack:

- A small handful of mixed nuts.

Day 4

Breakfast:

- Scrambled eggs with spinach and a side of whole-grain toast.

Lunch:

- Chickpea and vegetable curry with brown rice.

Dinner:

- Baked chicken breast with steamed green beans and quinoa.

Snack:

- Sliced cucumber with tzatziki sauce.

Day 5

Breakfast:

- Smoothie bowl topped with fresh berries, granola, and a drizzle of honey.

Lunch:

-   Mixed greens salad with grilled tofu, cherry tomatoes, and balsamic vinaigrette.

Dinner:

-   Baked cod with sautéed spinach and wild rice.

Snack:

-   Sliced bell peppers with guacamole.

Day 6

Breakfast:

-   Cottage cheese with sliced peaches and a sprinkle of sunflower seeds.

Lunch:

-   Spinach and kale salad with grilled chicken, cranberries, and a lemon tahini dressing.

Dinner:

-   Turkey and vegetable stir-fry with quinoa.

Snack:

- A small bowl of mixed berries.

Day 7

Breakfast:

- Whole-grain toast with smashed avocado and a poached egg.

Lunch:

- Minestrone soup with a side of mixed greens.

Dinner:

- Grilled tilapia with roasted Brussels sprouts and brown rice.

Snack:

- Sliced pear with cottage cheese.

Day 8

Breakfast:

- Green smoothie with spinach, banana, pineapple, and a scoop of protein powder.

Lunch:

- Quinoa salad with diced mango, black beans, red onion, and lime-cilantro dressing.

Dinner:

- Grilled turkey burger with a side of steamed asparagus and sweet potato wedges.

Snack:

- Sliced bell peppers with tzatziki sauce.

Day 9

Breakfast:

- Greek yogurt parfait with mixed berries and a drizzle of honey.

Lunch:

- Lentil and vegetable stir-fry with tofu and brown rice.

Dinner:

- Baked cod with sautéed kale and quinoa.

Snack:

- Sliced cucumber with hummus.

Day 10

Breakfast:

- Overnight oats made with rolled oats, almond milk, chia seeds, and topped with sliced strawberries.

Lunch:

- Spinach and arugula salad with grilled shrimp, cherry tomatoes, and balsamic vinaigrette.

Dinner:

- Chicken and vegetable curry with cauliflower rice.

Snack:

- A small handful of trail mix (nuts, seeds, and dried fruits).

Day 11

Breakfast:

- Scrambled eggs with diced bell peppers and a side of

whole-grain toast.

Lunch:

- Mixed greens salad with grilled chicken, cranberries, and a lemon-tahini dressing.

Dinner:

- Baked salmon with roasted broccoli and wild rice.

Snack:

- Sliced pear with almond butter.

Day 12

Breakfast:

- Smoothie bowl topped with fresh mango, granola, and a drizzle of honey.

Lunch:

- Chickpea and vegetable stir-fry with tofu and brown rice.

Dinner:

- Grilled tilapia with sautéed spinach and quinoa.

Snack:

- Carrot and celery sticks with guacamole.

Day 13

Breakfast:

- Cottage cheese with sliced peaches and a sprinkle of sunflower seeds.

Lunch:

- Minestrone soup with a side of mixed greens.

Dinner:

- Turkey and vegetable stir-fry with brown rice.

Snack:

- A small bowl of mixed berries.

Day 14

Breakfast:

- Whole-grain toast with smashed avocado and a poached egg.

Lunch:

- Spinach and kale salad with grilled chicken, dried cranberries, and a lemon-tahini dressing.

Dinner:

- Grilled chicken breast with roasted Brussels sprouts and quinoa.

Snack:

- Sliced apple with almond butter.

CHAPTER THREE

Lymphatic Diet Breakfast Recipe

1. Green Detox Smoothie

Ingredients:

- 1 cup spinach leaves
- 1/2 cucumber, peeled and sliced
- 1/2 avocado
- 1/2 banana
- 1 tsp chia seeds
- 1 cup unsweetened almond milk

Instructions:

1. Blend all the ingredients until smooth.

2. Pour into a glass and enjoy.

Cooking Time: 5 minutes

2. Overnight Chia Pudding

Ingredients:

- 3 tbsp chia seeds
- 1 cup unsweetened coconut milk

- 1/2 tsp vanilla extract
- 1/2 cup mixed berries

Instructions:

1. Mix chia seeds, coconut milk, and vanilla extract in a bowl.

2. Refrigerate overnight.

3. Top with mixed berries before serving.

Cooking Time: Overnight (5 minutes of prep)

3. Veggie Omelette

Ingredients:

- 2 eggs
- 1/4 cup diced bell peppers
- 1/4 cup diced tomatoes
- 1/4 cup chopped spinach
- Salt and pepper to taste
- Cooking spray

Instructions:

1. Whisk eggs in a bowl and season with salt and pepper.

2. Heat a non-stick pan, add cooking spray.

3. Pour in the whisked eggs.

4. Add veggies on one half of the omelette.

5. Fold the other half over the veggies.

6. Cook until set and serve.

Cooking Time: 10 minutes

4. Greek Yogurt Parfait

Ingredients:

- 1 cup Greek yogurt
- 1/4 cup granola
- 1/2 cup mixed berries
- 1 tbsp honey

Instructions:

1. Layer Greek yogurt, granola, and mixed berries in a glass or bowl.

2. Drizzle honey on top.

3. Serve chilled.

Cooking Time: 5 minutes

5. Quinoa Breakfast Bowl

Ingredients:

- 1/2 cup cooked quinoa
- 1/4 cup sliced almonds
- 1/2 sliced banana
- 1 tsp honey
- 1/4 tsp cinnamon

Instructions:

1. Mix cooked quinoa with sliced almonds.

2. Top with banana slices.

3. Drizzle honey and sprinkle cinnamon.

4. Serve warm.

Cooking Time: 15 minutes (for quinoa cooking)

6. Berry and Spinach Smoothie Bowl

Ingredients:

- 1 cup spinach leaves
- 1/2 cup mixed berries
- 1/2 banana
- 1/4 cup unsweetened almond milk
- 1 tbsp chia seeds
- Toppings: sliced strawberries, granola, and shredded coconut

Instructions:

1. Blend spinach, mixed berries, banana, almond milk, and chia seeds until smooth.

2. Pour into a bowl and top with strawberries, granola, and coconut.

Cooking Time: 5 minutes

7. Avocado Toast with Poached Egg

Ingredients:

- 1 slice whole-grain bread
- 1/2 ripe avocado

- 1 poached egg

- Salt and pepper to taste

Instructions:

1. Toast the whole-grain bread.

2. Mash the avocado and spread it on the toast.

3. Top with the poached egg.

4. Season with salt and pepper.

Cooking Time: 10 minutes (including poaching the egg)

8. Berry Protein Pancakes

Ingredients:

- 1/2 cup oat flour

- 1 scoop vanilla protein powder

- 1/2 tsp baking powder

- 1/2 cup mixed berries

- 1/2 cup unsweetened almond milk

- 1 egg

Instructions:

1. Mix oat flour, protein powder, and baking powder in a bowl.

2. Add berries, almond milk, and egg. Stir until well combined.

3. Heat a non-stick pan and pour in the batter to make pancakes.

4. Cook until bubbles form on the surface, then flip and cook the other side.

5. Serve with more berries on top.

Cooking Time: 15 minutes

9. Peanut Butter Banana Smoothie

Ingredients:

- 1 banana
- 2 tbsp peanut butter
- 1 cup unsweetened almond milk
- 1 tbsp honey
- 1/2 tsp cinnamon

Instructions:

1. Blend banana, peanut butter, almond milk, honey, and cinnamon until smooth.

2. Pour into a glass and enjoy.

Cooking Time: 5 minutes

10. Fruit and Nut Oatmeal

Ingredients:

- 1/2 cup rolled oats
- 1 cup unsweetened almond milk
- 1/4 cup mixed dried fruits and nuts (e.g., raisins, cranberries, almonds, walnuts)
- 1 tsp honey
- 1/2 tsp vanilla extract

Instructions:

1. Combine oats and almond milk in a saucepan.

2. Cook over low heat, stirring, until oats are creamy and cooked.

3. Stir in mixed fruits, nuts, honey, and vanilla extract.

4. Serve hot.

Cooking Time: 10 minutes

Lymphatic Diet Lunch Recipe

1. Lymphatic Detox Salad

Ingredients:

- 2 cups mixed greens (spinach, kale, arugula)
- 1/2 cup diced cucumber
- 1/2 cup cherry tomatoes, halved
- 1/4 cup grated carrots
- 3 oz grilled chicken breast (or tofu for a vegetarian option)
- 1 tbsp olive oil and lemon dressing

Instructions:

1. Combine mixed greens, cucumber, cherry tomatoes, and grated carrots in a bowl.

2. Top with grilled chicken (or tofu).

3. Drizzle with olive oil and lemon dressing.

Cooking Time: 10 minutes (if chicken needs to be cooked)

2. Lentil and Vegetable Soup

Ingredients:

- 1 cup green or brown lentils
- 1 onion, chopped
- 2 carrots, diced
- 2 celery stalks, chopped
- 4 cups vegetable broth
- 1 tsp cumin
- 1/2 tsp turmeric
- Salt and pepper to taste

Instructions:

1. In a large pot, sauté the onion, carrots, and celery until softened.

2. Add lentils, vegetable broth, cumin, turmeric, salt, and pepper.

3. Simmer for about 20-25 minutes until lentils are tender.

4. Serve hot.

Cooking Time: 30-35 minutes

3. Chickpea and Avocado Wrap

Ingredients:

- 1 whole-grain wrap
- 1/2 avocado, mashed
- 1/2 cup chickpeas, drained and rinsed
- 1/4 cup diced bell peppers
- 1/4 cup diced cucumber
- 2 tbsp hummus
- Handful of mixed greens

Instructions:

1. Lay the whole-grain wrap flat.

2. Spread mashed avocado and hummus on the wrap.

3. Add chickpeas, bell peppers, cucumber, and mixed greens.

4. Roll up the wrap and slice in half.

Cooking Time: 10 minutes (if chickpeas need to be cooked)

4. Quinoa and Black Bean Salad

Ingredients:

- 1 cup cooked quinoa
- 1 cup canned black beans, drained and rinsed
- 1/2 cup corn kernels (fresh or frozen)
- 1/4 cup diced red onion
- 1/4 cup chopped fresh cilantro
- Juice of 1 lime
- Salt and pepper to taste

Instructions:

1. In a large bowl, combine cooked quinoa, black beans, corn, red onion, and cilantro.

2. Drizzle with lime juice and season with salt and pepper.

3. Toss well and serve.

Cooking Time: 15 minutes (if quinoa needs to be cooked)

5. Mediterranean Tuna Salad

Ingredients:

- 1 can (5 oz) tuna in water, drained
- 1/2 cup diced cucumber
- 1/4 cup cherry tomatoes, halved
- 2 tbsp Kalamata olives, pitted and sliced
- 2 tbsp feta cheese
- 1 tbsp extra virgin olive oil
- 1 tsp lemon juice
- Fresh basil leaves for garnish (optional)

Instructions:

1. In a bowl, combine tuna, cucumber, cherry tomatoes, olives, and feta cheese.

2. Drizzle with olive oil and lemon juice.

3. Garnish with fresh basil leaves if desired.

Cooking Time: 10 minutes

6. Turkey and Vegetable Stir-Fry

Ingredients:

- 4 oz lean ground turkey
- 1 cup mixed stir-fry vegetables (broccoli, bell peppers, snap peas)
- 1 tbsp low-sodium soy sauce
- 1 tsp ginger, minced
- 1 clove garlic, minced
- 1/2 tsp sesame oil
- 1/2 cup cooked brown rice

Instructions:

1. In a wok or large skillet, brown the ground turkey over medium heat.

2. Add minced ginger and garlic, then stir in the mixed vegetables.

3. Add soy sauce and sesame oil, stirring until the veggies are tender.

4. Serve over cooked brown rice.

Cooking Time: 15 minutes

7. Spinach and Quinoa Stuffed Bell Peppers

Ingredients:

- 2 bell peppers, halved and seeds removed
- 1 cup cooked quinoa
- 1 cup chopped spinach
- 1/2 cup diced tomatoes
- 1/2 cup black beans, drained and rinsed
- 1/4 cup diced red onion
- 1/4 cup shredded mozzarella cheese (optional)
- Salt and pepper to taste

Instructions:

1. Preheat your oven to 375°F (190°C).

2. In a bowl, mix quinoa, chopped spinach, diced tomatoes, black beans, and red onion.

3. Season with salt and pepper.

4. Stuff the halved bell peppers with the quinoa mixture.

5. Top with shredded mozzarella cheese if desired.

6. Bake for about 25-30 minutes or until peppers are tender.

Cooking Time: 30-35 minutes (including baking time)

8. Grilled Salmon Salad

Ingredients:

- 4 oz grilled salmon fillet
- 2 cups mixed greens
- 1/4 cup cherry tomatoes, halved
- 1/4 cup sliced cucumbers
- 2 tbsp balsamic vinaigrette dressing

Instructions:

1. Place the grilled salmon on a bed of mixed greens.

2. Add cherry tomatoes and sliced cucumbers.

3. Drizzle with balsamic vinaigrette dressing.

Cooking Time: 10 minutes (if salmon needs to be grilled)

9. Sweet Potato and Lentil Bowl

Ingredients:

- 1 medium sweet potato, diced
- 1/2 cup cooked green or brown lentils
- 1/4 cup diced red onion
- 1/4 cup chopped fresh parsley

- 2 tbsp tahini

- 1 tbsp lemon juice

- Salt and pepper to taste

Instructions:

1. Roast diced sweet potatoes in the oven until tender.

2. In a bowl, combine cooked lentils, diced

 red onion, and chopped fresh parsley.

3. Whisk together tahini, lemon juice, salt, and pepper.

4. Serve the roasted sweet potatoes on top of the lentil mixture and drizzle with the tahini dressing.

Cooking Time: 30-35 minutes (including roasting sweet potatoes)

10. Quinoa and Kale Bowl with Lemon-Tahini Dressing

Ingredients:

- 1 cup cooked quinoa

- 2 cups chopped kale

- 1/4 cup diced red bell pepper

-   1/4 cup shredded carrots

-   2 tbsp tahini

-   Juice of 1 lemon

-   Salt and pepper to taste

Instructions:

1. In a bowl, combine cooked quinoa, chopped kale, diced red bell pepper, and shredded carrots.

2. Whisk together tahini, lemon juice, salt, and pepper to make the dressing.

3. Drizzle the dressing over the quinoa and kale mixture.

Cooking Time: 15 minutes (if quinoa needs to be cooked)

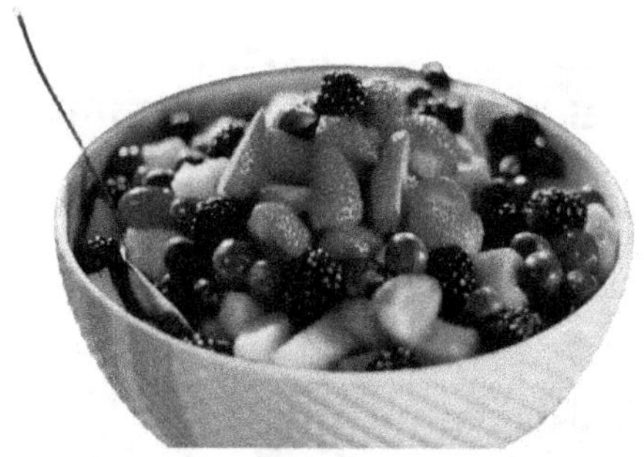

CHAPTER FOUR

Lymphatic Diet Dinner Recipe

1. Baked Salmon with Garlic and Herbs

Ingredients:

- 2 salmon fillets (6 oz each)
- 2 cloves garlic, minced
- 1 tsp dried thyme
- 1 tsp dried rosemary
- 1 tsp olive oil
- Salt and pepper to taste
- Sliced lemon for garnish

Instructions:

1. Preheat the oven to 375°F (190°C).
2. Place salmon fillets on a baking sheet.
3. In a small bowl, mix minced garlic, dried thyme, dried rosemary, olive oil, salt, and pepper.
4. Rub the garlic and herb mixture onto the salmon.
5. Bake for about 15-20 minutes or until salmon flakes easily.
6. Garnish with lemon slices before serving.

Cooking Time: 20-25 minutes

2. Quinoa-Stuffed Bell Peppers

Ingredients:

- 4 bell peppers, any color
- 1 cup cooked quinoa
- 1/2 cup black beans, drained and rinsed
- 1/2 cup corn kernels (fresh or frozen)
- 1/4 cup diced red onion
- 1/4 cup diced tomatoes
- 1/4 cup shredded cheddar cheese (optional)
- Salt and pepper to taste

Instructions:

1. Preheat your oven to 375°F (190°C).

2. Cut the tops off the bell peppers and remove the seeds.

3. In a bowl, mix cooked quinoa, black beans, corn, red onion, diced tomatoes, and shredded cheddar cheese (if desired).

4. Season with salt and pepper.

5. Stuff the bell peppers with the quinoa mixture.

6. Place the stuffed peppers in a baking dish and cover with foil.

7. Bake for about 30-35 minutes or until peppers are tender.

Cooking Time: 35-40 minutes

3. Lymphatic Detox Soup

Ingredients:

- 1 onion, chopped
- 2 carrots, diced
- 2 celery stalks, chopped
- 2 cloves garlic, minced
- 1 tsp turmeric
- 1 tsp ginger, minced
- 4 cups vegetable broth
- 1 cup kale, chopped
- 1 cup cooked chickpeas
- Salt and pepper to taste
- Fresh parsley for garnish

Instructions:

1. In a large pot, sauté chopped onion, carrots, celery, and minced garlic until softened.

2. Stir in turmeric and minced ginger.

3. Add vegetable broth and bring to a boil.

4. Reduce heat, add chopped kale and cooked chickpeas, and simmer for about 15-20 minutes.

5. Season with salt and pepper.

6. Garnish with fresh parsley before serving.

Cooking Time: 30-35 minutes

4. Grilled Chicken with Lemon-Garlic Asparagus

Ingredients:

- 2 boneless, skinless chicken breasts
- 1 bunch asparagus, trimmed
- 2 cloves garlic, minced
- Zest and juice of 1 lemon
- 1 tsp olive oil
- Salt and pepper to taste

Instructions:

1. Preheat the grill to medium-high heat.

2. Season chicken breasts with minced garlic, lemon zest,

olive oil, salt, and pepper.

3. Grill chicken for about 6-8 minutes per side or until cooked through.

4. Toss asparagus with lemon juice, salt, and pepper.

5. Grill asparagus for about 3-4 minutes, turning occasionally, until tender.

6. Serve grilled chicken with lemon-garlic asparagus.

Cooking Time: 20-25 minutes

5. Lentil and Vegetable Stir-Fry

Ingredients:

- 1 cup cooked green or brown lentils
- 2 cups mixed stir-fry vegetables (broccoli, bell peppers, snap peas)
- 4 oz firm tofu, cubed (or lean protein of your choice)
- 1 tbsp low-sodium soy sauce
- 1 tsp ginger, minced
- 1 clove garlic, minced
- 1/2 tsp sesame oil
- Cooked brown rice for serving

Instructions:

1. In a wok or large skillet, brown the tofu (or protein of your choice) over medium-high heat. Set aside.

2. Add minced ginger and garlic to the skillet, then stir in the mixed vegetables.

3. Add cooked lentils, tofu, soy sauce, and sesame oil, stirring until the veggies are tender.

4. Serve over cooked brown rice.

Cooking Time: 15-20 minutes

6. Lemon and Herb Quinoa with Roasted Vegetables

Ingredients:

- 1 cup cooked quinoa
- 2 cups mixed roasted vegetables (e.g., bell peppers, zucchini, cherry tomatoes)
- Zest and juice of 1 lemon
- 1 tbsp olive oil
- 1 tsp dried oregano
- Salt and pepper to taste

Instructions:

1. Preheat your oven to 400°F (200°C).

2. Toss mixed vegetables with olive oil, dried oregano, salt, and pepper.

3. Roast vegetables for about 20-25 minutes or until tender.

4. In a bowl, combine cooked quinoa, lemon zest, lemon juice, and roasted vegetables.

5. Stir well and serve.

Cooking Time: 30-35 minutes (including roasting time)

7. Spinach and Kale Salad with Grilled Shrimp

Ingredients:

- 8 oz grilled shrimp
- 2 cups mixed greens (spinach, kale, arugula)
- 1/4 cup cherry tomatoes, halved
- 1/4 cup sliced cucumber
- 2 tbsp balsamic vinaigrette dressing

Instructions:

1. Place grilled shrimp on a bed of mixed greens.

2. Add cherry tomatoes and sliced cucumber.

3. Drizzle with balsamic vinaigrette dressing.

Cooking Time: 15 minutes (if shrimp needs to be grilled)

8. Turkey and Vegetable Stir-Fry

Ingredients:

- 4 oz lean ground turkey
- 1 cup mixed stir-fry vegetables (broccoli, bell peppers, snap peas)
- 1 tbsp low-sodium soy sauce
- 1 tsp ginger, minced
- 1 clove garlic, minced
- 1/2 tsp sesame oil
- Cooked brown rice for serving

Instructions:

1. In a wok or large skillet, brown the ground turkey over medium heat.

2. Add minced ginger and garlic, then stir in the mixed vegetables.

3. Add soy sauce and sesame oil, stirring until the veggies are tender.

4. Serve over cooked brown rice.

Cooking Time: 15-20 minutes

9. Mediterranean Tuna Salad

Ingredients:

- 1 can (5 oz) tuna in water, drained
- 1/2 cup diced cucumber
- 1/4 cup cherry tomatoes, halved
- 2 tbsp Kalamata olives, pitted and sliced
- 2 tbsp feta cheese
- 1 tbsp extra virgin olive oil
- 1 tsp lemon juice
- Fresh basil leaves for garnish (optional)

Instructions:

1. In a bowl, combine tuna, cucumber, cherry tomatoes, olives, and feta cheese.

2. Drizzle with olive oil and lemon juice.

3. Garnish with fresh basil leaves if desired.

Cooking Time: 10 minutes

10. Grilled Veggie and Quinoa Bowl

Ingredients:

- 1 cup cooked quinoa
- 1 cup mixed grilled vegetables (e.g., eggplant, zucchini, bell peppers)
- 4 oz grilled chicken breast (or tofu for a vegetarian option)
- 2 tbsp tahini
- Juice of 1 lemon
- Salt and pepper to taste

Instructions:

1. Place cooked quinoa in a bowl.

2. Top with mixed grilled vegetables and grilled chicken (or tofu).

3. Whisk together tahini, lemon juice, salt, and pepper to

make the dressing.

4. Drizzle the dressing over the bowl.

Cooking Time: 20-25 minutes (if chicken or tofu needs to be grilled)

Lymphatic diet snacks recipe

1. Mixed Berry Smoothie

Ingredients:

- 1/2 cup mixed berries (strawberries, blueberries, raspberries)
- 1/2 banana
- 1/2 cup unsweetened almond milk
- 1 tsp honey (optional)
- Ice cubes (optional)

Instructions:

1. Blend mixed berries, banana, almond milk, and honey (if using) until smooth.

2. Add ice cubes if you prefer a colder smoothie.

3. Pour into a glass and enjoy.

Preparation Time: 5 minutes

2. Cucumber and Hummus

Ingredients:

-   1 cucumber, sliced
-   2-3 tbsp hummus

Instructions:

1. Wash and slice the cucumber.

2. Serve with hummus for dipping.

Preparation Time: 5 minutes

3. Greek Yogurt with Berries

Ingredients:

-   1/2 cup Greek yogurt
-   1/4 cup mixed berries (strawberries, blueberries, raspberries)
-   1 tsp honey (optional)

Instructions:

1. Spoon Greek yogurt into a bowl.

2. Top with mixed berries.

3. Drizzle with honey if desired.

Preparation Time: 5 minutes

4. Sliced Apple with Almond Butter

Ingredients:

- 1 apple, sliced
- 2 tbsp almond butter

Instructions:

1. Slice the apple.

2. Serve with almond butter for dipping.

Preparation Time: 5 minutes

5. Carrot and Celery Sticks with Hummus

Ingredients:

- Carrot sticks
- Celery sticks
- Hummus for dipping

Instructions:

1. Wash and cut carrot and celery sticks.

2. Serve with hummus for dipping.

Preparation Time: 5 minutes

6. Trail Mix

Ingredients:

- 1/4 cup mixed nuts (almonds, walnuts, cashews)
- 2 tbsp mixed seeds (pumpkin seeds, sunflower seeds)
- 2 tbsp dried fruits (raisins, cranberries)

Instructions:

1. Combine all ingredients in a small container.

2. Portion out as needed for a quick snack.

Preparation Time: 2 minutes

7. Sliced Bell Peppers with Guacamole

Ingredients:

- Sliced bell peppers (red, yellow, or green)
- Guacamole for dipping

Instructions:

1. Wash and slice bell peppers.

2. Serve with guacamole for dipping.

Preparation Time: 5 minutes

8. Cottage Cheese with Sliced Peaches

Ingredients:

- 1/2 cup cottage cheese
- 1/2 ripe peach, sliced
- 1 tsp honey (optional)

Instructions:

1. Spoon cottage cheese into a bowl.

2. Top with sliced peaches.

3. Drizzle with honey if desired.

Preparation Time: 5 minutes

9. Nut Butter and Banana Wrap

Ingredients:

- 1 whole-grain wrap
- 2 tbsp nut butter (almond, peanut, or cashew)
- 1 banana, sliced

Instructions:

1. Lay the whole-grain wrap flat.

2. Spread nut butter evenly on the wrap.

3. Place sliced banana on top.

4. Roll up the wrap and slice into bite-sized pieces.

Preparation Time: 5 minutes

10. Caprese Skewers

Ingredients:

- Cherry tomatoes
- Fresh mozzarella balls
- Fresh basil leaves

-   Balsamic glaze (optional)

Instructions:

1. Thread a cherry tomato, mozzarella ball, and fresh basil leaf onto a toothpick or skewer.

2. Drizzle with balsamic glaze if desired.

Preparation Time: 5 minutes

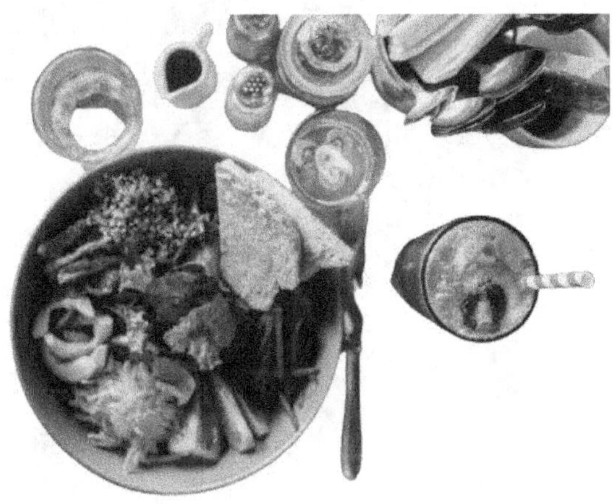

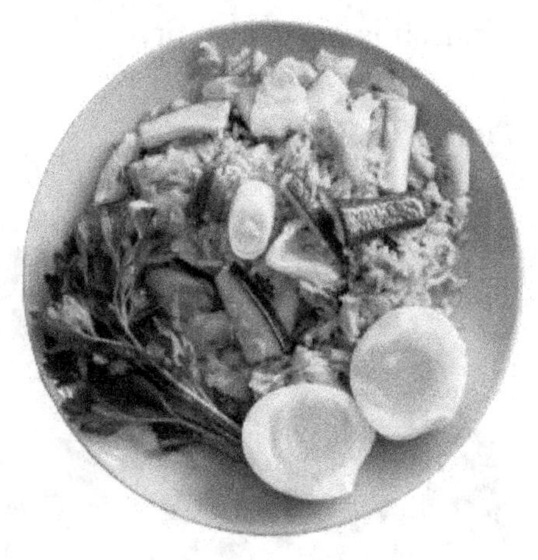

CONCLUSION

In conclusion, the lymphatic diet is a nutrition plan that emphasizes foods and practices aimed at supporting the lymphatic system's health and function. As a crucial component of the immune system, the lymphatic system plays a vital role in maintaining overall health and well-being.

By adopting a lymphatic diet, individuals can potentially enhance their immune responses, reduce inflammation, and promote efficient waste removal within the body.

The key principles of a lymphatic diet involve consuming foods rich in antioxidants, vitamins, and minerals, such as fresh fruits and vegetables. These foods help combat free radicals and reduce oxidative stress, which can contribute to lymphatic congestion.

Additionally, the diet encourages hydration through adequate water intake, ensuring that the lymphatic system operates optimally.

Furthermore, incorporating lean proteins, healthy fats, and whole grains into the diet provides essential nutrients for overall health while supporting lymphatic function. Avoiding processed foods, excess salt, and sugary beverages is also recommended, as they can contribute to lymphatic congestion and inflammation.

Meal planning is a critical aspect of the lymphatic diet, with balanced and nutritious meals being the cornerstone of its success. The lymphatic diet can be adapted to various dietary preferences, including vegetarian and vegan options, making it accessible to a wide range of individuals.

In conclusion, the lymphatic diet offers a holistic approach to health, focusing on nourishing the body's lymphatic system to support immunity, reduce inflammation, and promote optimal well-being.

By making mindful dietary choices and adopting a health-conscious lifestyle, individuals can harness the power of nutrition to improve their overall health and enhance the performance of their lymphatic system.

As with any dietary plan, it's essential to consult with a healthcare professional or registered dietitian before making significant dietary changes to ensure it aligns with individual health goals and needs.

www.ingramcontent.com/pod-product-compliance
Lightning Source LLC
Chambersburg PA
CBHW050855260726
48660CB00006B/2644